14 Day Palate Cleanse

Paula C. Henderson

ISBN-13: 978-1546457718

ISBN-10: 1546457712

CONTENTS

DISCLAIMER

ABOUT THE AUTHOR

Paula C. Henderson is a Nutritionist, Weight Loss Counselor and Author who makes her home in Las Vegas, Nevada.

Creator of the 5pts Free Diet which promotes easing your symptoms from auto-immune, inflammation, depression, insomnia, obesity, hypothyroid, menopause, arthritis and more through diet and a healthy lifestyle.

The 5 Points Diet Plan focuses on fresh foods you find in your local grocery store. Everyone is unique and this diet is customized to help you achieve optimal health and feel your best. #5ptsfreediet is dairy free, nightshade free, gluten free, soy free and grain free.

Paula grew up in Illinois and then moved to Ohio where, as a single mother, raised her daughter.

Becoming a certified weight loss counselor started an interest in healthy food choices and a healthy lifestyle that continues today. Taking care of one's self is even more important when facing daily challenges. Through the years Paula has continued her education as a Nutritionist and health care advocate.

Paula has written several books on diet and nutrition. By following Paula you will get a notification as she releases each new book.

www.amazon.com/author/paulachenderson

OTHER WORKS BY PAULA C. HENDERSON

A Gluten and Dairy Free, Grain Free, Soy Free, and Nightshade Free Grocery List: This is What's Left To Eat"

Paperback edition ISBN: 1542622727
Paperback details at: http://amzn.to/2oPfRGD

Kindle Edition: http://amzn.to/2nuCqQu

All You Can Eat Free Foods: Vegetables, Meats, Seafood and Beverages Grocery List

Paperback edition: ISBN: 1543155278
Paperback details at: http://amzn.to/2ofiPml

Kindle Edition: http://amzn.to/2oSUV1b

Tips For Your Weight Loss Success

Paperback edition: ISBN: 1539143457
Paperback details at: http://amzn.to/2oVvn0a

Kindle Edition: http://amzn.to/2phsS7U

Dictionary of Cooking Terms: For the Beginner Cook

83 basic cooking terms for the beginner cook, Safe Temps for Cooking Meats, basic preparation of common foods and an expanded bonus chapter of cooking tips.

Kindle Edition: http://amzn.to/2oPcfo1

Lettuce Amaze You: 100% Dairy, Gluten, Soy, Nightshade and Grain Free Lettuce Recipes

Paperback Edition: ISBN: 1540874931
Paperback details: http://amzn.to/2oTtlkh

Kindle Edition: http://amzn.to/2oT91PM

How I Got Free Stuff To Sell Online and Quit My Job

Paperback edition ISBN: 1542880653
Paperback details: http://amzn.to/2oTsjot

Kindle Edition: http://amzn.to/2oW2CAG

My Medical Information: A Log Book

Log your prescriptions, doctor visits, emergency room visits, eye doctor and dental visits, keep a list of your procedures, tests, and X-rays and more. Great if you need a caregiver and don't want to share online passwords or PIN to phone or laptop records.

Paperback edition ISBN: 1544058292
Paperback details: http://amzn.to/2nRG8Pp

Kids Prayer Request Book: Vacation Bible School and Sunday School

Paperback edition ISBN 1544960204
Paperback details: http://amzn.to/2oPGFGM

Prayer Request: Large Print Edition

These are a subtle gray and black cover rather than the traditional pink and flowery. Perfect for men and men's prayer groups or those who simply want another color choice. Also the large print is great for those with vision problems and those with a handicap that require larger spaces to write.

Paperback edition ISBN: 1544774176
Paperback details: http://amzn.to/2oPtHst

Incident Log Book: Stalking, Harassment and Domestic Abuse

Paperback log book ISBN 154501406X
Paperback details: http://amzn.to/2oTyyIT

1 WHY SHOULD YOU DO A 14 DAY PALATE CLEANSE?

I want you to crave what your body needs.
Not what it has become addicted to.

Touch your tongue to the top of your mouth. You are touching your palate. The palate is located in the roof of the mouth. It allows you to taste the flavor of foods, much like your taste buds on the back of your tongue.

Years of eating processed foods, sugary foods, artificial ingredients, too much sodium and preservatives dulls the palate. This is why so many people think vegetables taste bland. In reality they do not. But your palate has been dulled and distorted over time. Popular diets fail in large part because they would have you believe you can have processed foods while dieting. Not true.

If you truly want to take control of your health you must eat healthy foods. What this means is to exclude processed foods. Stay with me here. Don't panic!

Sure, we all have processed foods we like. But there are probably some foods that are not processed that you like too. Right? What are they? As you read through the chapters of approved foods start a list of the foods you like.

For those of you who are anxious about going 14 days without any processed foods I would suggest a short transitional period first. Here are some tips for the month leading up to your 14 Day Palate Cleanse:

- Stop eating dessert. Start weening yourself from the sugar if you add it to your tea or coffee. Just use a little less every few days or so. If right now you use two packets of sweeteners then go for a full week using a packet and a half. Then, try just a packet for the next week, then just a half a packet.

- Start choosing water as your beverage with all of your meals.

- Eat slower. Chew each bite more. I cannot stress this enough. Eat slower even if it means you do not have time to finish all of your food.

- Stop eating when you are full. Don't worry that you have left a bite or two on your plate. It's just a bite or two. Leave it. If you want to put it away for another meal, fine. But do not eat it if you feel full. If it's a vegetable or meat rinse it off or drain it if it has broth, sauce or gravy. Cut it into bite size pieces if it is not already in that condition. Place in the refrigerator to add to a vegetable soup later in the week, or the freezer for a soup next week.

- If you have a soda habit start weening yourself as with the sugar.

- Stop eating cold cereal, pasta, breads, desserts, granola and protein bars. Stop drinking juice. Stop eating frozen dinners.

- Eat out less if at all during this time.

- Don't try to reinvent the wheel. In other words eat foods in a way you already like them rather then trying to recreate a bad food into a healthy one. For example, don't try to figure out a way to prepare sweet potato pie. Just don't eat it. If you want a sweet potato, a whole, unprocessed food, eat it baked with unsalted real butter. Instead of trying to figure out an alternative for sugar just avoid sweets during this time. Choose savory foods that you already know you like. Go through the list in this book and circle the foods you like.

- If you don't already eat lettuce start experimenting with different ones. Find a few that you like. Remember that lettuce does not have to be chopped up into a bowl with dressing poured on it. Cut a wedge of iceberg lettuce, rinse it with cold water. Drizzle with a little oil, salt and pepper. Now pick it up with your hands and take a bite. Yes, like you would a celery stalk. As you rid yourself of the processed foods in your life this will start to taste much better and will not seem bland at all. Trust me. You can do the same with a Romaine Leaf. Pull off a stalk, rinse, etc. Eat like you would a stalk of celery. Some people enjoy drizzling lettuce with oil and vinegar and that's fine. Not a bottled dressing, but a healthy oil, and apple cider vinegar. You will read more about that later in Chapter six (6).

- Starting a **Banned Foods** List will go a long way toward building your self-discipline. When you add a food to your Banned Food List take it seriously and do not eat it. Not even in moderation. You have banned it from your diet. It is very important to start with one food you feel confident you can omit, but that you currently eat. This will make you feel more in control as you successfully commit to the Banned Food List that you create. As an example: my first banned food back in the 90s was donuts. This was a food I never bought at the store myself but they showed up at work, meetings, church, gatherings as I am sure they do for you as well. I always ate one. I felt it was okay since I never bought them to take home so I was just eating them "in moderation" when they showed up somewhere else. This was a food I felt I could successfully stop eating. *I banned it*! Perhaps your first Banned Food will be pancakes, or cookies or French fries. Once you feel you have successfully conquered that first food, add another. Perhaps potato chips or milk shakes. I observed early on in my journey that overweight people make statements like, "everything in moderation". Whereas, fit people make statements like, "I never eat that. I stopped eating that years ago." Banning a food or "eating in moderation" can make the difference in a healthy you or an unhealthy you.

- Start saying no to the extras like cheese, sour cream, bottled dressings, pickles, ketchup, desserts, sweets, snacks and second helpings.

- Eat when you are hungry. Stop eating AS SOON AS YOU ARE FULL. And do not eat if you are not hungry. Do not eat more than you need. Let me repeat that in a different way: Only eat what you need. No more.

The following chapters are a list of approved foods for your 14 Day Palate Cleanse.

This 14 Day Palate Cleanse will be: Gluten Free, Dairy Free, Soy Free, Nightshade Free and Grain Free.

Write your 14 consecutive days on your calendar like a countdown: 14, 13, 12, 11 and so on. If you have a day where you consume a food that is not approved simply start over: 14, 13, 12…. And continue until you have successfully gone 14 consecutive days eating only these approved foods.

Don't be discouraged if you find it takes many tries over several months. The majority of people are not able to do this the first try. Know that with each try you are that much closer to success and you have had that many more nutritious meals than you would have had eating before and it is that many less processed foods than you otherwise would have consumed.

Optimal effort will give you optimal results .

If you can continue on past the 14 days please do. A 45 Day Cleanse is optimal.

2 BEVERAGES

Water.

Try to remember this is temporary. For your optimal results of this Palate Cleanse you should only consume plain water. Don't worry, I have some solutions for you if you still are not in love with plain water.

If you MUST: have your caffeine in the morning at least limit it to a minimum and consume your caffeine within the first two hours you are up. After that stick to water. I could write an entire book on how good this is for you. Just consuming water. I will tell you that when I first started reading about healthy eating habits and read that one of the best things you could do for yourself, for your body, for your health was to limit beverages to simply water I could not imagine doing that. I just could not imagine only drinking water and nothing else. And yet, here I am loving it.

Things you can do to make your water more interesting and keep to the Palate Cleanse:

Carbonate it!

Add lime, lemon or orange slices are great added to water. Squeeze the slice first into your water then drop it in. Great for cold drinks and even hot water! You can even add the minimum amount of Raw, Unfiltered Honey if you feel you need it sweetened. But, I encourage you to avoid sweetener on a daily basis.

What about cucumber water?

- Peel and slice one medium to large cucumber into a GLASS pitcher. Fill with ice. Then with water. Cover. Put this in the refrigerator and allow the water to steep for at least two hours before servings. Fresh mint is especially good or lemon and lime slices really add to this water.

Fresh mint added to your water is very good! Again, as a cold beverage or as a hot mint tea. Get a mint plant and keep it on your counter.

Any other fresh herb that you like can be added to your water for flavoring or to make a nice cup of warm tea. www.gardeningknowhow.com is an excellent resource for brewing, growing, freezing and drying fresh herbs for tea and for cooking.

- Lavender
- bay leaf (yes)
- lemon balm
- lemongrass
- Ginger: go to your produce department and buy a ginger root. Simply store it in the freezer in a freezer bag. Slice off what you need, as needed, for tea and cooking.

It is best to avoid tea bags or loose leaf tea during the cleanse. The reason is the possibility of mold issues. Stick to the fresh herbs, fruits and vegetables to make your teas and beverages during your cleanse.

3 FRUIT

During this 14 Day Palate Cleanse I want you to limit fruit to breakfast and what tiny amount you may use for a beverage, squeezed over a salad or seafood.

- Do not place fruits in a juicer. No juicing. And you are to avoid all fruit juice of any kind. No juice.

Fruit: Do not assume all fruits are listed. Please read the list.

Reference the list when you are making out your weekly menu's and grocery lists. These should be eaten fresh from your local produce department or farmers market. Not dried, canned or frozen unless otherwise stated.

- **Apple**:   Best eaten whole, raw. An apple can also be sliced in a saucepan with a small bit of water as if to poach with a small amount of honey, cinnamon and nutmeg. This would make a nice, warm breakfast. For a sour apple choose green. For a sweet apple, choose a Gala apple.
- **Apricots**: As with the apple the apricot is good raw as is! It is also quite good poached for a warm breakfast.
- **Blackberries**: Berries are among the healthiest fruits and they are also among the lowest in sugars (carbs). Buy fresh berries of your choice, wash and remove stems. Spread on a baking sheet and set in the freezer for about an hour. Transfer to a freezer bag. Frozen blackberries are perfectly fine to purchase so long as the ingredient list is just blackberries. Toss various types of berries together in a

freezer bag to make your own breakfast mix. Blackberries, blueberries, cranberries, tart or sour cherries, raspberries and throw in a small handful of nuts and seeds. Berries are small enough that you can just pop them in your mouth straight from the freezer and are very refreshing especially on hot summer mornings.

- **Blueberries**: As with the blackberries. Fresh or frozen.
- **Cantaloupe**: Melon, like berries are of the lowest of the fruits for natural sugar content. So if you are watching your weight berries and melons are your best bet but still, watch your portions.
- **Capers** (In a jar. Drain and rinse before using) Generally used in savory dishes. My favorite is a Chicken Piccata. Poached chicken breast with capers, lemon juice, garlic served over fresh spinach.
- **Cherries** (tart or sour only. Not sweet or Bing cherries. There is a difference. Only fresh tart cherries from the produce department. These can be frozen, so if you find them on sale buy a few bags)
- **Clementine's** [citrus: If you occasionally experience RLS (restless leg syndrome, or, Overactive Bladder please avoid citrus during this time]
- **Coconut**: fresh only. Not the shredded in the bag.
- **Cranberries**: Fresh only. These freeze well. Simply put into a freezer bag. So buy when you find them on sale.
- **Grapes** (may be frozen. Eat sparingly as grapes are high in sugar!) These are a nice addition to your frozen berry mix. I find the purple and red taste very good frozen but the green not so much. For a treat: Combine purple grapes with a little water in your blender until smooth. Freeze in ice cube trays or popsicle molds.
- **Honeydew melon**: Fresh honeydew melon is an excellent choice as part of a low sugar, low carb breakfast.
- **Kiwi**: These are a great source of Vitamin C and fiber. A frequently asked question is whether or not the skin is edible: Yes, it is!
- **Lemons** [citrus: If you occasionally experience RLS (restless leg syndrome, or, Overactive Bladder please avoid citrus during this time]
- **Limes** [citrus: If you occasionally experience RLS (restless leg syndrome, or, Overactive Bladder please avoid citrus during this time]
- **Mango** (very high carb so eat minimally if you are trying to lose weight)
- **Muskmelon**
- **Nectarine** [citrus: If you occasionally experience RLS (restless leg syndrome, or, Overactive Bladder please avoid citrus during this

time]

- **Oranges** [citrus: If you occasionally experience RLS (restless leg syndrome, or, Overactive Bladder please avoid citrus during this time]
- **Papaya** [high carb, eat sparingly]
- **Peach:** Another fruit I think is best fresh but a tasty warm breakfast option when poaches.
- **Pear:** There are several varieties of pears and they each have their own distinct taste. Mix it up and try them all!
- **Pineapple:** these really are not as difficult as one would think to cut. I have a hard time with some squash and some root vegetables and yet have never had a problem with a fresh pineapple. Can also be frozen for a nice treat! Or, added to water. Do not juice your pineapple, but you could put some pineapple in your blender with a bit of water and blend for a smoothie textured drink. If you catch them on sale buy several, go ahead and cut up. Spread on a baking sheet and freeze for one hour. Transfer to freezer bags.
- **Plum:** Plums are a nice way to mix it up on occasion. Eat when in season.
- **Pomegranate:** At least try one!
- **Raspberries:** Fresh or frozen. If you purchase frozen, be sure the ingredient list is raspberries, and only raspberries.
- **Strawberries:** Need we say more?
- **Watermelon:** Watermelon is a delightfully hydrating fruit! So refreshing and your body loves foods that are high in water content. I like to make a watermelon salsa:

Chop watermelon and toss with fresh chopped cilantro, oil, white onion, salt, pepper and a splash of lime juice to taste. Best after allowed to sit in the refrigerator for at least an hour, covered tightly and always in a glass bowl. Salsa is also excellent made with cucumber this same way.

4 VEGETABLES

Do not assume all vegetables are listed. Please read the list..

- **Acorn Squash**: If this guy is too difficult to cut in half raw try boiling it for about 30 minutes first. Then, cut in half, drizzle with oil, salt and pepper and then bake at 375 for another half hour.
- **Artichoke**: Fresh or canned. If you use canned be sure to drain and rinse well. Have you had artichoke dip? Sometimes referred to as artichoke hummus?

1 14 ounce can artichoke hearts, packed in water, drained
1 clove garlic, minced
2 Tbsp. extra virgin olive oil, or another healthy oil you like. I have been using a Sunflower/Avocado Blend Oil.
1 Tbsp. fresh lemon or lime juice
¼ cup tahini or sesame oil
¼ tsp. ground cumin
Salt and pepper to taste
Fresh herbs such as parsley or cilantro, minced

- **Arugula**: Just 8 calories in 2 cups! If you are looking to add a peppery kick to your salad or dish try the peppery tasting Arugula. Makes a nice bed for your grilled steak, fish or chicken breasts. Always toss with oil, salt and pepper and vinegar if you like it when using as a bed for your meat, seafood or other vegetables.
- **Asparagus**: Best way to enjoy your asparagus is toss fresh or frozen asparagus with oil, salt and pepper. A tiny bit of garlic powder is fine but it really does not need it. Spread evenly on a baking sheet. Bake at 400 degrees for 15-20 minutes or until tender.

Best when it has turned a bit charred or golden brown so hit it with the broiler if it didn't.

- **Avocado**: Well too many recipes for the avocado so I will share my most common way to enjoy it. Chop into a bowl, add chopped, fresh cilantro. Toss with oil, apple cider vinegar, salt and pepper.
- **Bamboo Shoots** (drain and rinse) One of the healthiest foods you will find. Use them in stir fry, soups and even in salads.
- **Basil** (fresh only) Keep a basil plant in the house. They smell wonderful and look pretty. Best of all when you use fresh herbs that you grow yourself. Picking just what you need as you need it allows the rest to stay on the plant and not wilt. If you need to trim your herb(s) you can freeze dry them for later use. Wash and spread onto a baking sheet, putting the baking sheet in the freezer for about an hour. Then, transfer to a freezer safe freezer bag.
- **Beets** (high sugar content! Eat sparingly)
- **Bibb Lettuce**: what a great lettuce to use as a lettuce wrap or lettuce cup. Use in place of taco shells for tacos, especially fish tacos! Bibb Lettuce can be more expensive in the grocery store. But you can easily grow bibb lettuce yourself at home outside or in a container.
- **Bok Choy**: A crunchy delightful vegetable with so many uses. Look up some recipes and try this healthy low carb veggie if you haven't.
- **Broccoli**: [exception a cruciferous. If you are hypothyroid you should only eat cruciferous vegetables cooked. Never raw.] An easy dairy free low carb creamy broccoli soup: chicken broth and cooked broccoli (fresh cooked or thawed frozen) in the blender until smooth. For a silky smooth you will have to blend it longer than it seems you should! Transfer to a saucepan to heat through adding salt and pepper. Garlic is especially good in this soup and some like to add a splash of lime juice or apple cider vinegar to add a brightness.
- **Brussels Sprouts** [exception a cruciferous. If you are hypothyroid you should only eat cruciferous vegetables cooked. Never raw.]
- **Butternut Squash** (high carb, eat sparingly)
- **Cabbage** [exception a cruciferous. If you are hypothyroid you should only eat cruciferous vegetables cooked. Never raw.]
- **Carrot**: Don't dismiss carrots as a boring run of the mill vegetable. We all agree they are nutritious but I encourage you to look for recipes and new ways to use these in your day to day cooking. I make a breakfast puree using 3 medium carrots, one small Gala Apple. Boil both until tender. Allow to cool. (I usually will boil the

night before). Add just part of the liquid, all of the carrots and apple to the blender and blend until smooth. Add honey, cinnamon and nutmeg to taste. Heat through.

- **Cauliflower** [exception a cruciferous. If you are hypothyroid you should only eat cruciferous vegetables cooked. Never raw.]
- **Celery**: A good source of flavor for many dishes, low carb and nutritious.
- **Chives**: Fresh only and easy to grow at home.
- **Cilantro**: Cilantro is very nutritious, low carb and you can use it for more than just salsa. Growing this herb yourself is easy but it is also available year round at affordable prices.
- **Collards**: Collard Greens are a great source of calcium, fiber and Vitamin C.
- **Crookneck Squash**: Low carb so great for any diet. A great side dish or main entrée. Sauté' with onion, raw with dip or boil and mash with butter and garlic.
- **Cucumber**: Very hydrating. Try to find the one without the wax so you can also eat the peel. Cucumber liquefies when added to your blender so it is the great start of a homemade salad dressing.
- **Dandelion**: A dark green leafy that is a good source of Vitamin C, magnesium and more.
- **Dill**: fresh only
- **Endive**: Such a beautiful lettuce. Great addition to other vegetables on a vegetable and dip tray.
- **Fennel**: If you are avoiding raw cabbage due to thyroid disease this is a nice substitute.
- **Garlic** (fresh garlic bulbs only. You can freeze garlic bulbs. Simply place in a freezer bag as is.)
- **Ginger Root** (fresh only) Also may be frozen as is. Simply place the root in a freezer bag. Keep on hand to make tea (hot and cold) and for cooking.
- **Green Beans**: Fresh green beans are nothing like canned or frozen. My favorite methods are tossing with oil, salt and pepper. Spread evenly on a sheet pan and bake at 400 for 20 minutes until browned. Another is to simmer in chicken broth and garlic in a skillet until tender.
- **Herbs**: all fresh herbs. Grow the ones that are too expensive at the store.
- **Horseradish**: jar or fresh. If you buy a jar of horseradish please read the ingredient list as all of the ingredients must be on this approved list. Avoid soybean oil, spices, and other unknown

ingredients. If you cannot find a jar of pure horseradish, purchase a horseradish root. You can freeze the root by just placing it in a freezer bag. Shave, grate or cut of as needed and return the root to the freezer).

- **Iceberg Lettuce**: For years we have heard, "iceberg is mostly just water". Yes it is and that's good news! We want water and it is terribly important to stay hydrated. Besides water lettuce is nothing but nutrients so nothing bad going on here. Such low carbs you can eat all you want. A refreshing, hydrating, low carb, low calorie, no fat, nutrient rich food? Count me in. Don't be afraid to just cut it into wedges and pick it up with your hands and eat like you would a stalk of celery.
- **Jicama**: a high carb root vegetable so go easy on the jicama
- **Kale** [exception a cruciferous. If you are hypothyroid you should only eat cruciferous vegetables cooked. Never raw.]
- **Kohlrabi**: taste like a combo of cabbage and turnips
- **Leeks**: be sure to clean leeks properly. If whole rinse under running water. If you will be preparing them chopped, place the chopped leeks in a bowl of water; allowing it to sit for a moment. Use your hand and shimmy the leeks in the water a bit. Using a slotted spoon remove the leeks from the water. It is suggested to repeat this to be sure all of the dirt has been removed.
- **Lettuce**: all varieties. Look around the next time you are in the produce department. There are many different varieties of lettuce and greens. Some are peppery, some are bitter, some are more sweet and water (a good thing!). So try them out and buy the one that suits what you will be using it for. I have included a chapter on the different lettuce varieties with a description later in the book.
- **Mushrooms** [exception: You should avoid mushrooms if you have been diagnosed with candida, or are vulnerable to getting yeast infections, hives, or athletes foot (a fungus)]
- **Mustard Greens**: pairs well with onions and garlic. Sauté the onions and garlic first, then add the mustard greens. Drizzle with apple cider vinegar, salt and pepper before serving.
- **Napa Cabbage** [Exceptions: a cruciferous. If you are hypothyroid you should only eat cruciferous vegetables cooked. Never raw.]
- **Okra**: Have you tried baking whole frozen okra? You must. Toss frozen whole okra with oil, salt and pepper. Spread onto a baking sheet. Bake in a 400 preheated oven until golden brown. About 10 minutes, turn the okra over or turn to broil and leave in another 5 or 10 minutes.
- **Olives**: drain and rinse. Black olives, Kalamata olives, and green.

Remove pimento from green olives. Pimento is a nightshade.

- **Onions**: keep onions on hand. They are healthy and a great way to season your foods. Research recipes and expand on onion use. Different onions are best for different dishes too. Red, yellow, white onions, scallions, leeks, shallots.

- **Parsley**: Fresh only. This is not just a garnish! And so very healthy. Parsley is very easy to grow but it is also really affordable at your local produce department in any store. Parsley has anti-inflammatory properties and helps with digestion and is known to strengthen the immune system. A great source of Vitamin C, A, E and potassium. Make chimichurri or salsa verde: 1 cup of fresh parsley leaves, 1 cup of cilantro (optional), diced white onion or scallions, oil, apple cider vinegar, salt and pepper. Best when allowed to sit for about 30 minutes before serving. Eat as a side, tossed in with other salad greens or to top fish, chicken, steak or a nice soup topping. Great way to get your daily vinegar.

- **Parsnip** (higher carb, eat sparingly)

- **Peas** (Green Peas: fresh or plain frozen peas) A good pairing is green peas with spaghetti squash!

- **Pumpkin**: canned pumpkin is ok, but be sure the ingredients list is just pumpkin and nothing else.

- **Radicchio**: Some people don't like radicchio because of its bitter flavor but grilling it mellows that. Drizzle with oil, salt and pepper and put it on the grill, or, you can put it in the oven at 400 until golden brown, about 10 minutes, or hit it with the broiler.

- **Radish**: The radish is a good source of your B vitamins and an excellent addition to almost any salad or vegetable tray.

- **Rhubarb**: Very healthy but resist preparing in the traditional way in desserts. There are quite a few savory rhubarb recipes out there that are quite tasty indeed.

- **Romaine Lettuce**: Everyone's favorite lettuce. Salads of course but do you cut it lengthwise, drizzle with oil, salt and pepper and roast in the oven or put it on the grill? How about adding to a vegetable tray, picking up with your hands like a stalk of celery and dipping? I have recently started using Romaine sliced in thin strips in place of raw cabbage for slaw because I am hypothyroid and want to avoid raw cruciferous.

- **Rutabaga** (high carb. Eat sparingly)

- **Sage** (fresh only) Have you tried Sage Butter?

- **Scallions**: Also known as Green Onions

- **Shallots**: More or less known as the mild onion.

- **Snap Beans**: Depending on what part of the country you are in a Snap Bean or a Green Bean.
- **Snow Peas**: The flat green bean you usually find in Asian dishes.
- **Sugar Snap Peas**: If you are not a fan of the Green Bean, try these!
- **Spaghetti Squash**: Most recipes state to cut this vegetable in half raw, place on a baking sheet and bake. I boil mine whole and then cut it in half. I find this much easier. Whichever you prefer this is a great, low carb vegetable that is quite versatile.
- **Spinach**: What can we say? Entire books have been written about the nutrition and versatility of this near perfect vegetable.
- **Squash**: Not all squash are created equal! Yellow Squash, Crookneck squash, Summer Squash and Spaghetti squash are great; eat all you want. Butternut, acorn, pumpkin are all types that are high in carbs much like the yam and sweet potato so eat those sparingly if at all if you are trying to lose weight.
- **Sweet Potato** (very high carb. Eat sparingly if at all while trying to lose weight)
- **Swiss Chard**: a lovely dark green leafy full of nutrients.
- **Tarragon** (fresh only)
- **Turnips**: If you haven't tried it, do. If you don't like them don't worry. Many don't For fans this can be used in lots of various dishes and offers many good health benefits.
- **Turnip Greens**: Taste nothing like the turnip of course. A vegetable all on their own.
- **Wasabi Root and Wasabi Peas**: Careful of the high carb content.
- **Water Chestnuts** (drain and rinse well)
- **Watercress**: A beautiful healthy leafy green.
- **Yellow Squash**: The yellow squash and the Zucchini are two of the lowest carb and nutrient rich foods you can eat.
- **Zucchini**: So many different ways to prepare zucchini and yellow squash. Not everyone likes both. So if you tried one and did not like it; please be sure to try the other. They do taste a bit different. My favorite preparation is to simply cut lengthwise, toss in oil, salt and pepper and grill or bake until tender and turning brown.

5 NUTS AND SEEDS

Not the ones in the snack aisle, but rather the ones in the baking aisle. The ingredients should just be the nut or seed. No salt, spices or dried fruits. No mixed nuts in a can. Nuts can be a culprit in weight gain. Yes, they are healthy, but they are fattening too. Limit your portion if you eat them at all.

Exceptions: Nut allergies of course, but if you are vulnerable to yeast infections, athletes foot, other fungus related flares or have been diagnosed with Candida try omitting all nuts and seeds from your diet much like someone with a peanut allergy would avoid nuts. Do this for a good solid month to see if your symptoms go away.

6 VINEGARS AND OILS

Leave your bottled dressings behind during your 14 Day Palate Cleanse. They are a processed food. Making your own dressings is quick and easy and you'll get the hang of it very quickly. You can also make it once for the week and keep it in a jar in the refrigerator if you don't have time to make it fresh each time you need it.

Oil:

- Avocado Oil
- Coconut Oil
- Grapeseed Oil
- Olive Oil
- Sunflower Oil
- Peanut Oil [exception: avoid if you are prone to candida, yeast infections, fungus, athletes foot]

Vinegar:

- EXCEPTIONS:

Avoid Malt Vinegar as this is a gluten.

Avoid store bought prepared salad dressing like Italian Vinegar and Oil, etc… Opt for pure vinegars during this time. You do not want added ingredients like *spices, acidic acid, citric acid, soybean oils, etc.

Any combination of these oils and the vinegar will make a nice dressing. Add salt and pepper, perhaps some fresh garlic, minced onion, or fresh herbs like basil, maybe lime juice instead of vinegar?

You can also use your vegetables to make a very nice dressing. Try peeling a cucumber and put it in your blender with some oil, a drizzle of vinegar, salt and pepper. Add avocado for a creamy texture. You can also make a dressing out of all things lettuce! Add about 1/8 cup oil to your blender and 1 cup chopped lettuce, a drizzle of vinegar or lime juice, salt and pepper. Blend until the lettuce has pureed. Garlic is a nice addition (after the blending). Store in frig for at least a few hours before serving or make the night before.

Raw Unfiltered Apple Cider Vinegar *"with the mother"* should also be on the label. Can readily be found in all grocery stores with the regular vinegar. Take this seriously as regular apple cider vinegar will not have the same positive health affects we are looking for.

During the cleanse I want you to consume at least 2 ounces of Raw, Unfiltered Apple Cider Vinegar every day. Ways to incorporate Raw Unfiltered Apple Cider Vinegar into your daily diet:

Drink a mixture of:
1 tablespoon raw honey
2 ounces of Raw, Unfiltered Apple Cider Vinegar
2 ounces of slightly warm water

Or you can make a salad dressing using the Raw Unfiltered Apple Cider Vinegar mixing a healthy oil, salt and pepper with as much of the vinegar as you can tolerate. Use as your salad dressing at lunch or supper or both. Or if not having salad, toss make a chimichurri or salsa verde tossing it with chopped parsley or cilantro to be eaten ahead of the meal or at minimum it should be the first thing you consume off your plate. You could also toss an avocado with your cilantro, onion or cucumber.

7 SWEETENERS

Raw Unfiltered Honey: take this seriously. Do not get just any honey you find. Raw Unfiltered Honey is different but it can be found in any grocery store with the regular honey. It should state Raw, Unfiltered on the front of the bottle or jar.

Please remember this is still a sweetener and should only be used sparingly. Omit completely if you can. For optimal results your Cleanse would not include any sugars. Avoid eating even natural sugars on a daily basis.

8 PROTEINS

Eggs: boiled or poached only
Lentils [Exception: due to the high carb value please limit consumption frequency and your portion size.]
Nuts: Although a healthy fat, a fat none the less so limit your portion.

Avoid cured meats:
- Lunchmeat
- Hot dogs
- Breakfast sausage
- Ham
- Bacon
- Italian sausage
- Polish sausage
- Bratwurst

Poultry, Beef, Pork and Seafood:

- Poultry: Whole chicken, hen, turkey. Ground turkey, ground chicken. Uncooked, unseasoned is what you are looking for. Bone in and skin on is what will give you a good stock or broth.
- Beef: Ground beef, steak, roast, ribs. Uncooked, unseasoned is what you are looking for. Bone in is what will give you a good stock or broth.
- Pork: Ground pork, pork chops, ribs. Unseasoned and uncooked is what you are looking for.
- Seafood: Raw, uncooked, unseasoned seafood that you cook and prepare at home is what you are looking for. If you are sensitive

to sodium please read packages as some seafood's do have higher amounts of sodium.

- Avoid canned meats and seafood during your cleanse.

If you eat meat at all limit your portion during this time. Meats should either be omitted or limited to just 25% of your food consumption.

- Never eat meat at lunch.
- Limit lunch to vegetables only.
- Limit fruits and nuts to breakfast.

Serve fish 3 times a week for your evening meal. You need not eat it any more often than 3 times a week but a minimum of three (3). Unbreaded. Baked, steamed or poached only. Season with herbs, vegetables or fruits. Eating an array of different kinds of fish is a good idea but if you only choose one or two please do not have tuna 3 times a week due to the possibility of mercury. Once in a while is certainly safe. Try cod, salmon, and other different types of seafood as well as tuna. Avoid canned if you can and eat fresh. It need only be a small portion as the largest part of your meal should be vegetables.

9 MISCELLANEOUS FOODS

- Unsalted Real Butter
- Arrowroot: Can be found in the area of the cornstarch generally. To be used in place of cornstarch and flour.
- Sea Salt (Preferably Iodized Sea Salt or Himalayan Salt) Most of us will want the iodized unless your physician has prohibited you from using an iodized sodium)
- Black Pepper: course, Restaurant Style Black Pepper is best.

10 PREPARATION AND STORAGE

Yes, how you prepare, what you prepare your foods in and how you store them does matter during your 14 Day Palate Cleanse. I would like to encourage you to adopt some, if not all, of these methods and continue them even after your cleanse period is over.

You may prepare the foods on this list in the following ways during your 14 Day Palate Cleanse:

- Poach: To simmer in a small amount of water. Unlike boiling, poaching is to merely simmer a food in a shallow amount of water.
- Boil: To cook food in boiling water whereas the food is usually covered completely in water.
- Bake
- Blanched: To add food to boiling water for a brief moment and then quickly removed.
- Steamed
- Raw

Store and prepare foods in glass whenever possible. Beverages and everything else. Personally I have arthritis and had replaced most of my heavy glass with plastic back in the 90s. Now, I am reverting back to glass and I am happy to find that there are much lighter versions out there. If you too have a problem with the weight of heavy glass dishware check around. There are still the very heavy brands but many brands are making a lighter version!

Invest in the Rubbermaid or Pyrex Red Top glass storage containers. A great buy and you will find that you use them daily.

Pyrex: Includes storage bowls with lids as well as the baking dishes http://amzn.to/2oPoAHJ
Rubbermaid Glass storage containers with lids: http://amzn.to/2ovCYRQ

Do not wash green leafy vegetables until you are ready to consume. Only wash the portion you will be consuming at the time of consumption. The reason for this is that fresh produce stays fresh longer by keeping it dry.

While you do not want to microwave foods in plastic containers it is perfectly fine to freeze them. Stick with BPA free plastic if you can, but freezer bags are also okay to use. It is the heat interacting with the plastic that is bad. According to eatingwell.com freezing foods renders bacteria inactive. So as long as you place foods in the freezer that were not originally contaminated, it will not become contaminated while frozen due to the plastic. Just be sure to use Ziploc bags specifically marked as freezer bags and containers that indicate they too are for freezing in order to prevent freezer burn.

You can also buy ball jars for storing some foods.

I have started to save glass jars and lids from olives, artichokes and vinegars. They can be washed and sterilized. Great for storing liquids, dressings, sauces and soups that you make. Also nice to store freeze dried herbs from your own herbs you grow at home or if you have dried them.

11 FAQ

Obvious omissions from this list: To be clear: I want you to AVOID these foods during your cleanse.

Avoid Legumes: with the exceptions of dried lentils. Not canned.

Avoid Nightshades:

Avoid all peppers, tomatoes, white and red potatoes, eggplant.

Avoid Grains:
- Corn
- Rice
- Oats
- Wheat (also a gluten)

Dried seasoning except salt and black pepper.

Soy Products: soybeans, edamame, soy sauce, soybean oil, soy milk.

Gluten: bread, pasta, whole wheat flour, bleached flour, crackers, etc.

Gluten Free breads, flour, cereal and pasta: all processed foods we want to avoid during a Palate Cleanse. Not because they are gluten free but because they are a processed food.

- All vegetables, fruits, nuts, seeds, meats and seafood are gluten free.

Avoid Dairy: All dairy with the exception of Unsalted Real Butter. Please only use unsalted real butter sparingly or omit completely.

Dairy Free alternatives like Almond milk except the smallest of amounts when necessary. No more than 8 ounces a day.

Sugar: white sugar, brown sugar, artificial sweeteners, syrup, and stevia. If you must have sweetener in your morning coffee or tea, try using raw, unfiltered honey and even then, use the minimum amount needed to still enjoy your coffee. All sweeteners, including honey, is a food you should have a goal of eliminating from the diet except on rare occasion. You should not make a practice of daily consumption. Try to begin weening yourself off it slowly if going cold turkey is not for you. Perhaps start weening yourself off the sugar a few weeks prior to doing your 14 day cleanse.

12 RESOURCES

http://www.fruitsandveggiesmorematters.org

http://www.livestrong.com

www.organicfacts.net

www.ingramcontent.com/pod-product-compliance
Lightning Source LLC
Chambersburg PA
CBHW071315280526
45788CB00004B/1901

* 9 7 8 1 5 4 6 4 5 7 7 1 8 *